The Violent Thief

The Violent Thief

A Young Girl's Story of Growing up with Her
Mentally Ill Mother

NANCY GRACE WILLIAMSON

Dedicated to my

wonderful and heroic parents

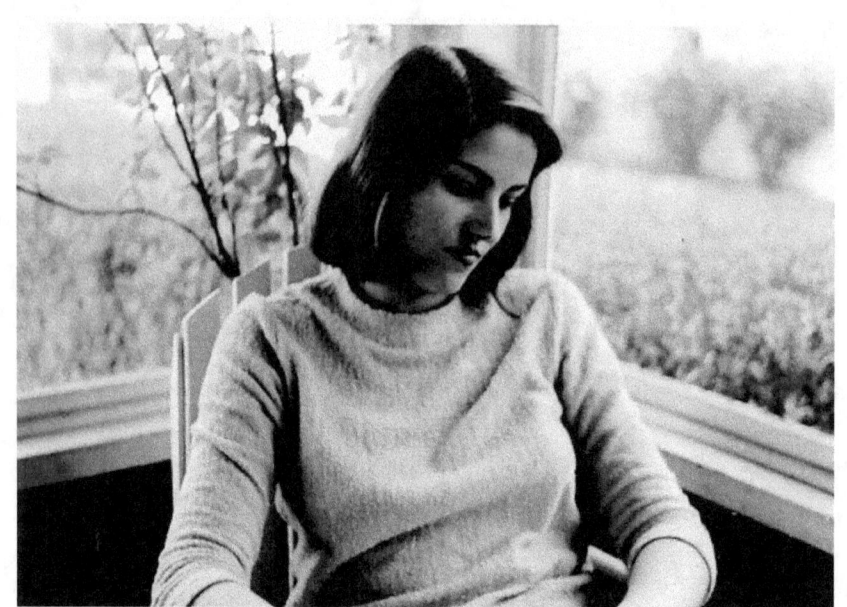

Introduction

I wrestled with the decision to write this book because I would be sharing some very personal and private things about my life and my family. As a registered nurse, I have seen the urgent need in our society to get up to speed in our understanding of mental illness. Not only do we need to be more educated about mental illness in general, but we also need to increase our research efforts so that we can better treat and eventually cure these plagues that steal so many lives. Additionally, we need to have a heightened awareness of what the families of the mentally ill are often called to endure. These reasons motivated me to share my story.

In many ways I feel as if my parents are writing this book with me. It is our story and our hope that those who struggle with mental illness will be met with more empathy and less judgment and that their families will be shown more compassion and understanding. May we learn to look for the people within the illness and not just for the illness itself.

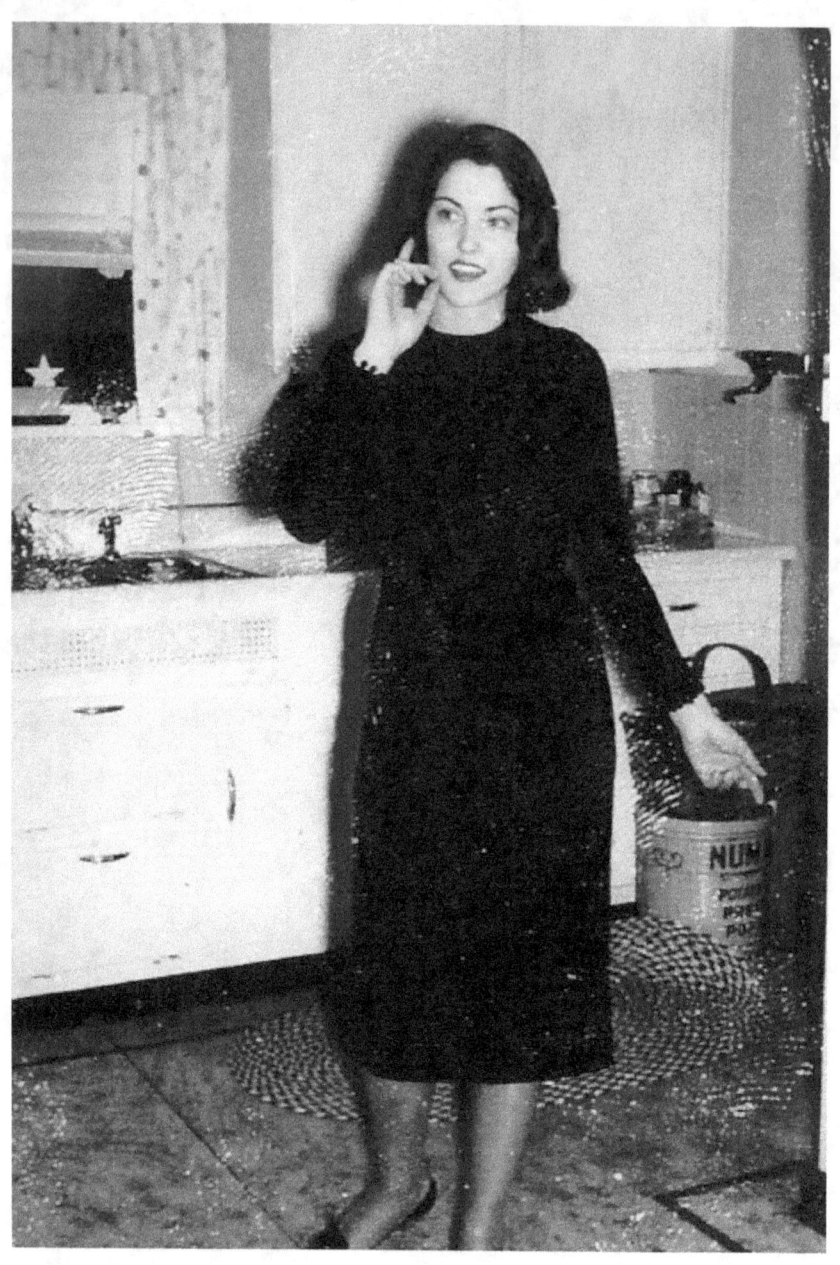

Carol at the Magee Street home.

CHAPTER 1

Simply put, she was beautiful. Her brown hair, her bright smile, and her beautiful eyes caught the attention of all the boys in her high school. Everyone knew Carol was the youngest daughter of the family that sold eggs out of their home in Lakewood, Ohio. The family was also known for running an egg and produce stand in the downtown Cleveland market. Many a boy looked forward to picking up the eggs from the family business with the hope that they would get to see beautiful Carol. If they were particularly lucky, they may even get the chance to talk to her.

But when it came to boys, Carol was very picky. When she would agree to a date with a boy, she made it very clear that she had high standards.

No kissing on the first date—or ever—if she wasn't feeling it. Her dating policy earned her the title with the high school boys as "frigid." They could call her what they wanted, and she didn't care. She was saving herself for that special someone who was most definitely in her bright future. She was waiting for that person she would settle down with, raise a family with. She looked forward to her happily ever after. People would say she had her head in the clouds, but she knew her life would be all that she hoped it would be.

Carol was a multi-talented girl. She swam, skied, played tennis, and was very active in her school. To hear her sing was a treat for people of all ages. She was asked to sing at many events and was considered to be an up-and-coming talent in the Cleveland area. She also had great taste in clothes. This simple girl from a simple family was voted "Best Dressed" in her class. Still, those who knew her best felt that her most notable qualities were her sweetness, her kindness, and her gentle soul. She also had a fantastic sense of humor.

Carol and her friends would often laugh until they peed in their pants.

I suppose it was the laughing that brought me back to reality. As I sat on the city bus over 30 years later, I looked to my left and wondered how this could be the same woman who did and felt all those things as a young girl. I looked at her face, so worn and confused. Her eyes were crazy looking, her clothes old and in need of replacement. But when you live disability check to disability check, there isn't extra money for new outfits.

I purposely sat on the outside seat when we took the city bus. It made me feel as though I could protect her better that way. Even though I was only fifteen years old, I somehow felt a lot older and bigger than I was. Would someone look at her funny on the bus today? Would someone make a comment when she would laugh out loud uncontrollably to herself to the point that tears would run down her face? Maybe someone would laugh at her when she would sit there and rattle off nonsense, sometimes arguing out loud with an imaginary person.

I was always ready to give an angry glare to anyone who would look at her in a disrespectful way. At the tip of my tongue sat the statement, *What's your problem? Can't you tell she has a mental illness? Leave her alone.* I would let no one hurt her that day or any day.

I knew who she really was inside even though no one else could see it. Little did all those people on the bus know that they were amongst greatness, beauty, intelligence, talent, and goodness. They didn't know who she was, but I did, and I loved her. I knew that she wanted to be present more than anything and that this illness was not her choice but a bad deal that life handed her. She suffered more than anyone I ever knew. This wonderful woman was locked up in a body that was her prison. It held her captive from all that life offered and all that she had looked forward to as a young girl. It held her captive from the one thing she wanted most: to be a mother. I could see and feel her pain. I knew it well because I was her daughter.

CHAPTER 2

It wasn't so bad being in her twenties and living at home with her parents. Carol's older siblings had moved out and were raising their own families, so for now, she was fine living at home. She and her mother, Lena, got along well, and she was always going to be daddy's little girl. Living at home also made it possible for Carol to help her parents take care of Uncle Wally, who lived with them. Wally lost his vision as a young boy after being blinded from shoveling snow. The slight vision he held onto was taken by glaucoma in his later years. Lena refused to put her brother in any type of care facility. Wally needed extra help ever since his stroke and Carol was happy to help out.

Like most young adults, Carol was finding her path in life. After trying college for a short period, she realized she was much happier when she was working and making money. She eventually found a great job as a legal secretary. She went to work dressed beautifully and always wore a big smile.

Carol's job paid well, enabling her to pursue her passion for travel. When she traveled, she loved bringing home gifts for her nieces. Once she brought them little matching cashmere sweaters. The girls were in awe! It was always a treat for Aunt Carol to visit because she loved giving gifts to those little girls.

Carol was also singing at many high-end clubs in Cleveland. After one particular performance, an agent approached her. As he handed her his card, he said he could make her a star. But after pursuing his offer, Carol found out that the agent wanted her to get a nose job before promoting her any further. Carol thought this was ridiculous and was not willing to alter her body for the small chance that the agent could further her career, so she continued to find her own singing gigs around the Cleveland area. Once she was asked to sing for the Christmas program in a famous music hall in downtown Cleveland. It was a high honor to perform at such a prestigious place.

Carol's social life was going well. She dated some great guys. She became serious with one man in particular and thought he could be the guy she had waited for and dreamed about as a little girl. He wanted to marry her too, but something just didn't feel right. Eventually, they broke up.

The breakup seemed to throw Carol into a tailspin. She became anxious and depressed and sought psychiatric counseling. The counselor told her she was too uptight and needed to loosen up. He recommended that she start drinking a little more alcohol in the evening to help her deal with her nerves. He prescribed medication and Carol started drinking and smoking more to deal with her mental condition. The counselor's advice infuriated Carol's mother, Lena. Now it was well known that Carol's family enjoyed their beer and alcohol—as most German families do—but for a counselor to encourage her daughter to take up such behavior seemed outrageous.

As Carol entered her late twenties, something peculiar happened. One day while at work, she looked at the sky and began to duck because she was worried the planes in the sky were going to hit her. Carol's work supervisor called Lena, and Lena took Carol home. Over the next few years, Carol was given shock treatments to help her cope with her increasing psychiatric problems. A new diagnosis was given: paranoid schizophrenia. Lena questioned this diagnosis. Did they really know what they were talking about? Was her psychotic episode a result of mixing medication and alcohol? What about all these shock treatments they were giving her? What lasting effect did they have on Carol? Lena felt resentment toward the mental health profession. After all, it was a mental health professional who told her daughter that more drinking would cure her. Lena and her husband, Bill, felt helpless as they watched their beautiful daughter's life unravel.

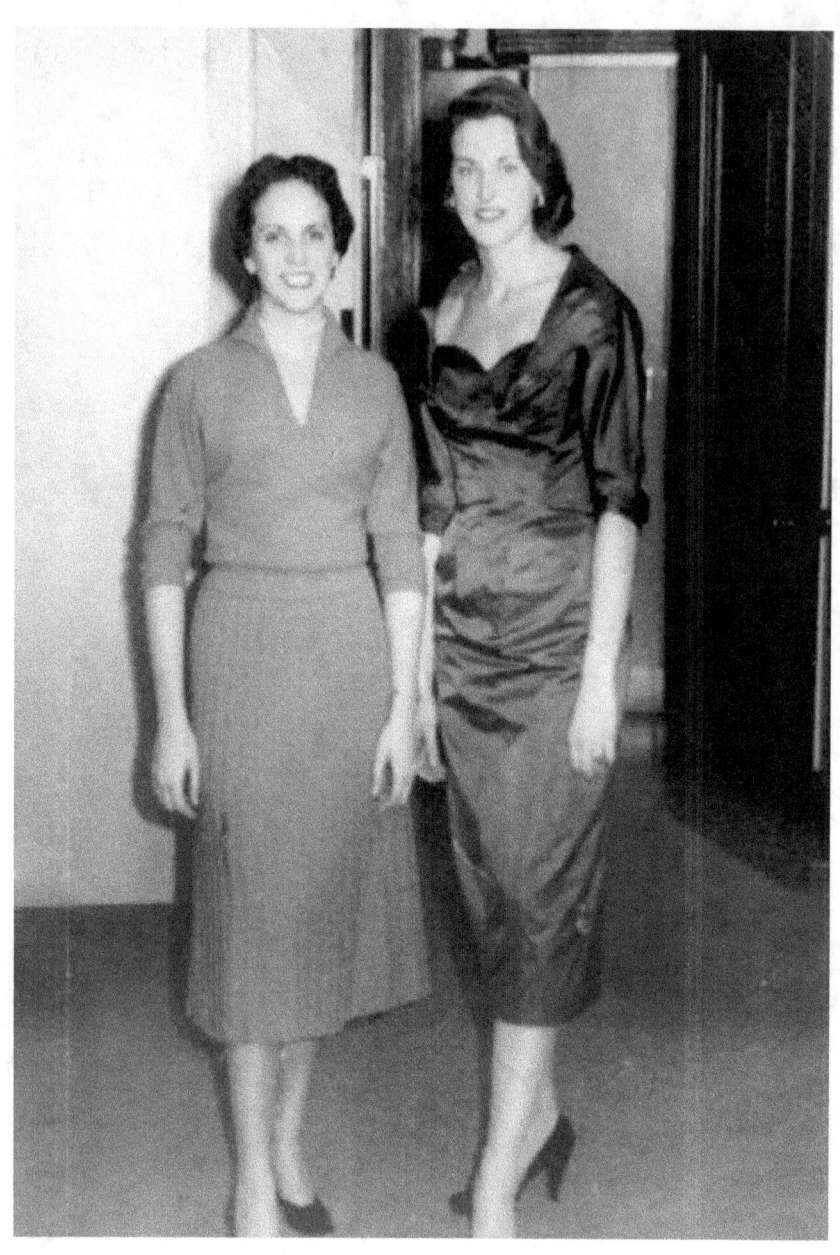

Carol (right) with her coworker.

CHAPTER 3

Over the next few years, Carol was prescribed stronger medications. During that time, her alcohol intake also increased. She entered her thirties still living at home. She went through good and bad periods. Her bad periods were usually due to her taking her medication inconsistently. She eventually lost her secretary job and began working for a temporary employment agency.

Carol continued to sing for nightclubs in Cleveland. During one of her good periods, she went on a date to a restaurant. They were enjoying a nice dinner when a strong redheaded man approached her at their dinner table. Ignoring her date, he looked at Carol and said, "You are the most beautiful woman I've ever seen. May I have your number?" Carol and her date looked at each other for a moment and said nothing. Carol reached into her purse, pulled out a pen, and scribbled her number onto a napkin and handed it to the man.

A few days later, she received a call from Dave, the bold Scottish man who had approached her at the restaurant. They spent the next few months enjoying each other's company. They both loved to sing and would record duets together on their tape recorder. Carol's signature song that she often showcased in nightclubs was "Climb Every Mountain." Now Carol and Dave sang this song together for their own enjoyment.

Carol's family did not approve of her new relationship. Her family valued hard work and industry above everything else, and Dave—a self-employed sign painter who lived paycheck to paycheck—didn't meet their expectations for what they had in mind for their daughter. Even though they knew she had her struggles, they didn't think he was the best fit for their beautiful Carol. They didn't approve of her dating a man who had been honorably released from the military with some PTSD symptoms. "What a disaster this could be," they thought.

Dave and Carol continued to date and enjoy each other's company. One day, at the age of thirty-two, Carol found out that she was pregnant. This came as a shock to both her and to Dave. A baby was not in the plans for either of them at this time in their lives. Nevertheless, they were both thrilled. When Carol approached her family with this unconventional news, they were concerned. Considering her struggles with mental health, one family member suggested that she should look into the possibility of putting their baby up for adoption. Carol and Dave would not hear of such a thing. In fact, the soon-to-be-mother already knew in her heart that she was going to have a little girl. She began buying clothes for her baby. Dave would ask her, "Why don't you buy some boy clothes? It could be a boy, you know." But she would always answer, "No, I know it's a girl." In light of her pregnancy, she stopped drinking and smoking and made a conscious effort to eat healthy food. Dave and Carol would go on walks together at night because they felt it was good for their baby's development.

A few months before the baby was due, Carol bought a nice pink knee-length maternity dress, and the couple went downtown to the Old Stone Church in Cleveland, and, without anyone knowing, they were married. They moved into an apartment together a few miles away from her family home and began their new life together.

On Carol's parents' wedding anniversary, Carol and Dave welcomed me into the world. They named me Nancy Grace. Carol was doing great both mentally and physically. Her mind seemed clear and healthy. She breastfed her baby and was an incredibly attentive mother. "You shouldn't pick up the baby every time she cries, or you will spoil her," Dave would say to his wife. But Carol disregarded his advice, and she was quick to soothe and to attend to me.

When I was a toddler, my parents' marriage became very rocky. Carol grew more anxious and the couple would fight. In the midst of their turbulent relationship, Carol received the heartbreaking news that her father had died suddenly of a heart attack. Soon after, Carol and Dave divorced. My mom and I moved back to her family home on Magee Street to live with her mother and her Uncle Wally.

The home on Magee Street held a lot of meaning and memories for the family. Lena, Carol, Wally, and now I lived in the house that Lena and Wally had spent their whole lives in. It was the very house that Lena and Wally's dad built when he emigrated from Switzerland. It went from being the base for their locally famous Swiss Dairy to the family business where they sold eggs. These days it was a simple home on a simple street across from a large factory on the border of Lakewood and Cleveland. It was the same home that Carol and her mother were born in; now it was the place where Carol would raise her daughter.

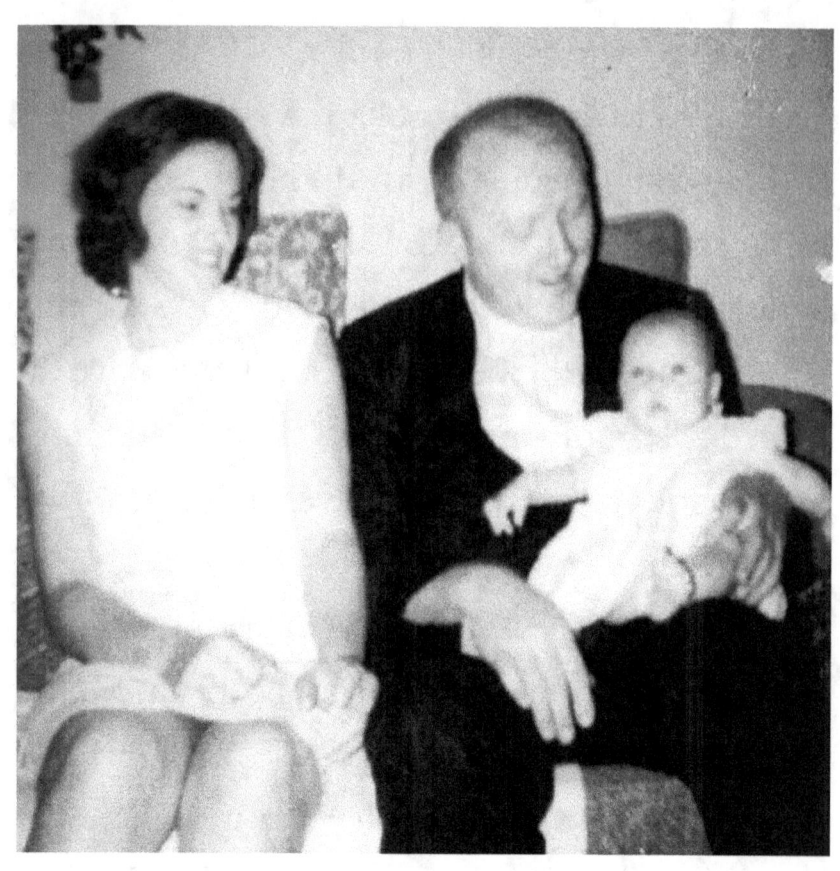

Carol, Dave, and Nancy.

CHAPTER 4

In spite of the divorce, Dave and Carol had an amicable relationship. They both loved their little girl and wanted the best for her. It was at this point that my dad, Dave, began a pattern that would continue throughout my growing years. He would come over every night for a few minutes to visit with me, and on Sundays, he would take me to visit my Scottish grandparents who lived in the Cleveland housing projects. Grandma Lena didn't let him come into the house, so he would visit on the porch or in the yard. He never missed a chance to see me.

As a little girl, one of my most favorite things was to have my mom read to me. My favorite was Snow White and the Seven Dwarfs. I loved hearing how the prince rescued the princess even after the mean witch tried to kill her. During my early years, my mom and I shared a bedroom and a bed in our two-bedroom house. I would line up my stuffed animals along the sides of the bed and curl up next to my mother while she read to me. This was our nightly routine. My mom read Snow White, and I would beg her to read it again and again, and she always happily obliged. The two of us would fall asleep under our blue bedspread surrounded by stuffed animals.

At one point, my mom tried to work again, and I was taken to a daycare center. My parents dropped me off for my first day at the center. After leaving me there for a few hours, my dad had a feeling that he should go back and check on me. He picked up my mom and they headed back to the daycare. When they walked back into the room, the nice-looking lady who greeted them was gone, and in her place was an elderly man whom my dad described as "crippled." This man was the only adult in the building and was sitting in a chair amongst a group of preschoolers. The crippled man asked my mom if she would tie his shoe. At that odd request, my dad frantically began looking for me and eventually found me laying in my cot for naptime. Strangely enough, I still remember that cot and how cold and sterile it felt. My dad snatched me up and the three of us left. After this incident, my parents never put me in daycare again. Instead, Grandma Lena cared for me while my mom attempted to work.

In spite of some odd circumstances, I felt happy and secure as a young girl. I was excited about life! I remember the magical feeling I had the night before my first day of school. I sat on the porch swing between my mother and my grandma and felt the warm, humid Ohio air on my skin. The next day, my dad took me to Harrison Elementary for my first day of kindergarten. He said he would stay with me for a while in the classroom, but I told him to leave because I was OK. He left with tears in his eyes.

During my elementary years, my mom wanted me to learn a skill, but because of her fragile mental health, it was very hard for her to take me to any type of class on a regular basis. At different times, I was enrolled in gymnastics, baton lessons, and tap dancing. Since I only attended each class a few times, I never actually learned to do any of those things.

My mother's love language was giving gifts. Despite the ups and downs of her schizophrenia and our low income, she always managed to buy me many thoughtful presents when I was young. I loved the smell of the Higbee Department Store bags, which held my Christmas presents. That was the most exciting smell in the world! Even though I knew Santa brought presents, I somehow understood that there was a lot of stuff for me in those Higbee bags! One year I peeked into one of the bags that was hidden in the closet. I happened to get a glimpse of a Baby Tender Love, a baby doll that I desperately wanted. I was thrilled on Christmas morning to find that Santa had somehow brought me the same doll that I saw hidden in the closet bag.

When I was in first grade, my mom threw me a big birthday party and invited a bunch of kids from my elementary school over to our home. She made a homemade piñata out of crepe paper and filled it with toys and candy. It was such a joyous and exciting day! I even wore my fancy blue jacket with gold buttons on it for the special occasion.

Shortly after the party, my mom began taking her medication inconsistently, and her illness grew worse. Her weight began to fluctuate a lot. She smoked cigarettes incessantly and seemed to have some strange obsession with the singer Tom Jones. While I was still a young girl, my mom took me to a Tom Jones concert. A few days after the concert, I watched as she grabbed all of the record albums in the house and threw them into the garbage in the backyard. She was swearing and saying something about Tom Jones as she dumped them into the garbage can. It was an odd thing to do, but it also felt somewhat normal. I began to see my mother exhibiting strange behaviors on a more consistent basis.

Despite my mother's bizarre behavior, I was always happy to be home. I loved my house, my family, and my community. I had a great group of friends to hang out with. Our neighborhood gang of kids was very active. We made a pet cemetery in our yard under my pine tree. All of my fish, hamsters, and guinea pigs that died were placed there. We also made room for some random guests that were found in the neighborhood: birds, frogs, and other little critters we found dead under trees and on the streets around our homes. My friends and I would always have a proper funeral service for our little pals who had gone to the great beyond. I would read something completely random from Grandma's Bible, and we would end our service by all saying "Amen." Soon we were off to a new adventure on our bikes or in a tree or somewhere in the neighborhood.

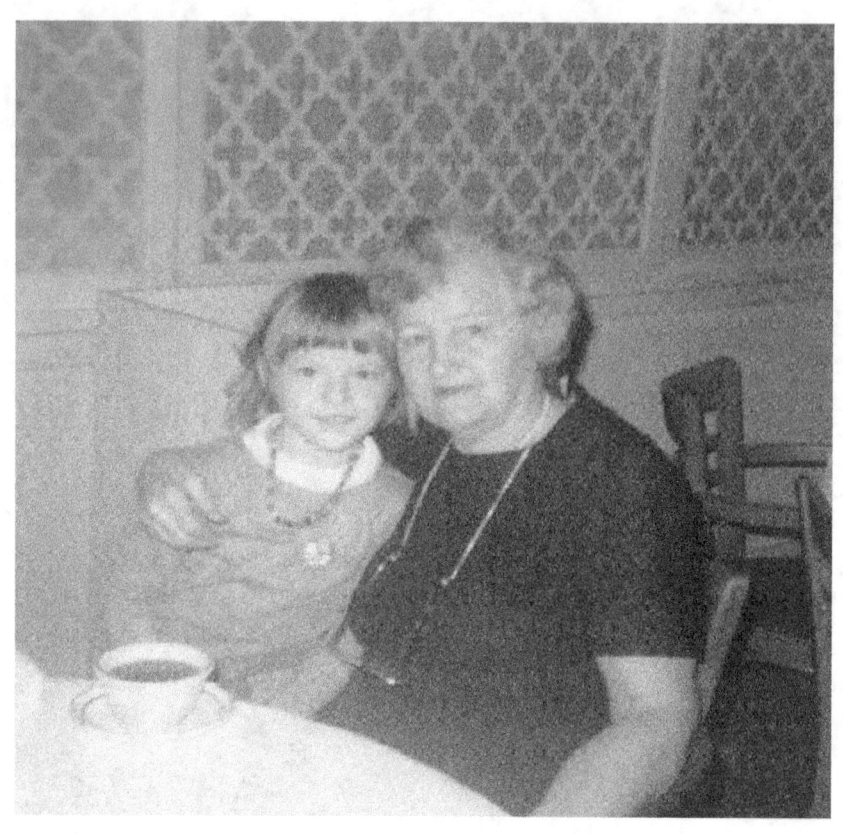

Nancy with her grandma.

Chapter 5

It was during my second-grade year when my mother's illness spiraled out of control. I must have started sensing that my mom's condition was getting worse because I began having nightmares about her hurting other people. Even though she was a sweet, gentle, and wonderful woman in her real and healthy state, my dreams reflected the change that I was seeing in her.

On the night before Easter, I had a very vivid dream. I saw my mother hurting my grandma. I woke up very agitated and angry. That Sunday morning my mom kept trying to convince me to put on my Easter dress and bonnet for church, but I refused any suggestion that she had that morning.

A few nights later, I became scared in the middle of the night and went to sleep in my grandma's bed. I continued to sleep there for the next five years. Our family dog, Cocoa, also slept in the bed with Grandma and I. I loved my dog, even though he would bite my feet if I moved too much during the night.

Sleeping in that room led to many great discussions between my grandma and me. One night, she asked me what I wanted to be when I grew up. I stated that I wanted to be a nurse. My grandma, being a straight shooter and being someone who was very much to the point, responded, "Good. Do that. You should be a nurse." In another one of our nightly conversations, my grandma randomly said, "One day you will go to college, and when you do, you should go to college in a different state. Do not stay here and go to school." I really didn't know what she was talking about or what she meant by her comment, so I just tucked it away in my brain for later.

My move into my grandmother's room must have been very painful for my mom as she struggled to keep herself together. She began to drink more and went off her medication again. From this point on, her deterioration seemed to accelerate. Grandma and I would often wake up in the middle of the night to the sound of my mom screaming in the kitchen while she was slamming cupboard doors. She would swear and scream at the top of her lungs. Grandma would go to the top of the stairs and yell down, "Stop that, Carol! What the hell are you doing?" When my grandma would climb back into bed, I would curl up next to her back and try to go to sleep. I felt safe when I was close to my grandma.

My mom just wanted to feel normal and healthy again, but she didn't know how to do that. One day, she decided to put an ad in the paper for someone to carpool with her to Las Vegas. On some level she must have been thinking, "I used to travel all the time. Taking a trip will help me feel better." Her condition had worsened to the point where she could no longer drive, so she asked for someone to drive her to Las Vegas and offered to help pay for gas. Sure enough, to my grandmother's horror, a random man answered the ad in the paper. My mom suddenly announced that she was leaving in a few days with this strange man. My grandma did everything she could to stop her, but nothing worked.

A red car pulled up in front of our house, and without any of us seeing the man's face, my mom opened the door and got in. My grandma, who couldn't move very quickly due to her arthritis, quickly instructed me to take the camera and run after the car as they drove away so we could get some pictures of the license plate. I ran alongside the car as it left, and as it slowed down to turn the corner, I snapped a bunch of pictures of my mother driving away with this stranger. I didn't understand the dangers of what she was doing, but I felt anxious that she was leaving with a man that no one knew.

My mom eventually returned two weeks later, seemingly without incident. No one really knew what happened on that trip. We just moved on with life and never spoke about it again.

My grandma was my anchor. She was the glue that held our family together. Somehow, this widow with arthritis did all the housework and laundry, paid the bills, did all the cooking, shopping, etc. In addition, she cared for her brother, her mentally ill daughter, and now she was raising me. She wasn't shy about having me work. She made me work a lot! Besides walking the dog every day, I would often spend a good part of my Saturdays dusting and vacuuming, trimming hedges, pulling weeds, and working in the yard. After a very long hot day of work, Grandma would drive me to the ice cream store where I was allowed to get a dipped ice cream cone. That was the payment. No money, no allowance, just an ice cream cone, and I was perfectly happy with that.

Grandma had her own way of handling life's problems. Cocoa hated the mailman and would jump on the screen door when he came to deliver the mail on the porch. One morning, Cocoa jumped on the locked door, opening the door, and bit the mailman in the testicles. We found out later that Cocoa's teeth had broken through the skin, and the mailman had to be treated by a doctor. There was no lawsuit and we never saw a medical bill. Instead, Grandma bought the mailman a case of Jack Daniels, and it was never spoken of again.

~

The more incapacitated my mother grew, the closer I became with my Gram. In the mornings, I would pick out my clothes for the school day, sit on the couch in the living room, and wait for Grandma to wake up. She would come down the stairs and braid my hair, and then I was ready to go on with the day. I walked to my elementary school and would walk home for lunch. Grandma always had a hot lunch waiting for me. Usually it was tomato soup and a grilled cheese sandwich. I found out later that my dad would often sit in his car and watch me walk to and from school without me knowing it. He was concerned about my safety in our declining neighborhood. Every night for dinner, Grandma prepared a hot meal. We ate a lot of sauerkraut, pork chops, liver, and potatoes. I loved it when she made homemade bread. There was nothing like a piece of her warm bread with butter on it. It made our whole house smell wonderful! Her apple Kuchens were to die for; my mouth would water just thinking about her moist, delicious sponge cake.

During that time, there was a TV show that would honor what they called "The Most Wonderful Woman in the World." On this show, the host would surprise a woman by reading her a letter that someone wrote about her and then present this woman with a great gift. I watched that show one day and then sat down and wrote a letter to submit. In my letter, I wrote that my grandma was "The Most Wonderful Woman in the World" to me and that I would appreciate it if the show would give her a trip to Switzerland because that is where she always wanted to go so she could see the land that her parents came from. I was too young to know where to send the letter, and it just seemed to disappear after I wrote it.

Our morning routine included getting Uncle Wally up from his twin bed in the living room. Someone in the family would dump out the urinal, which was usually full from the night, and then we would stand him up with the walker and dress him. Next, we would walk him to the kitchen to his rocking chair where he would spend the day. When it was time to eat, we would also move him to the table. When he needed to go to the bathroom, we would stand him up and walk him to the commode, set him down on the pot, then if needed wipe him when he was done. We spent many years repeating this routine. No one ever complained. We loved Uncle Wally. In spite of his blindness, paralysis from his stroke, and decreased hearing, there wasn't a senile bone in his body. As long as you spoke loudly, he always knew who was talking to him and what was going on.

The kitchen was usually a happy place. All seemed to be well in the world when our family of four sat and enjoyed a warm meal together. For that small moment, problems seemed to go away. Even Cocoa was happy since Uncle Wally loved to share his food by throwing scraps to him under the table.

~

One morning, I woke up and heard a lot of yelling. I raced downstairs and found my mom standing over my grandma, who was sitting at the kitchen table. My mom had a crazy look in her eyes and was yelling things that didn't make sense. I could instantly tell that this was *not* my mom. This was the other person, the crazy person, who showed up that morning for whatever reason. My mom was holding my grandma's hand in hers and was yelling and shaking the elderly woman's arm and fingers. My heart was pounding. I immediately put myself between my mom and grandma and pushed my mother back, yelling at her to stop. Finally, my mom released Grandma's arm. Again, this was *not* my mother. This was her illness, the sick version of herself. Grandma, who was always a pillar of strength, was crying and very shaken up. This experience intensified my fear that one day something bad may happen to my grandma.

Shortly after this incident, we went to visit my grandpa's grave at the cemetery. I overheard Grandma say, "When I die . . .," and then it dawned on me that one day my grandma would die. After all, she was an older woman and old people died. From that point on, I began praying every night that God would never let my grandma die. I also prayed that He would not let my mother, father, or Uncle Wally die either. I said that prayer every night for many years.

Living with a mentally ill mother always made life unpredictable. There were more than a few times when the police forcibly took my mom to the mental hospital. I wasn't sure why she was taken away, but I was sad that I would not be able to see her. One time, I followed the policemen out of the house as they escorted her to the police car and asked the officer, "Can I go too?" The officer coldly told me to "go back into the house with your grandma."

My mom went through short periods of appearing stable. She had a job for a while at Burger King. None of her job attempts lasted very long, and this one was no exception. While at work, she would start talking to herself, then suddenly laugh out loud uncontrollably. Understandably, this made the customers and the other employees very uncomfortable, never mind the fact that she could not focus on what she was doing. Sometimes she would spontaneously leave work and walk home. One day she was fired on the spot and sent home.

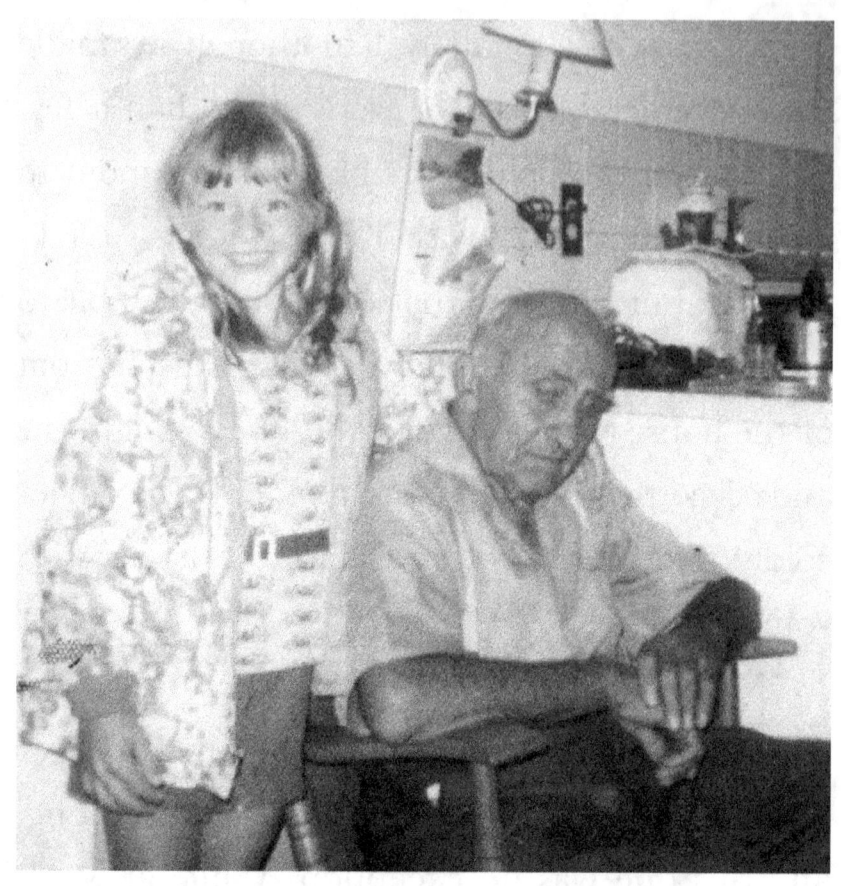

Nancy with Uncle Wally.

CHAPTER 6

Even though my mom's illness was consuming, there were a lot of very healthy things in our life. My parents went together to my parent-teacher conferences for most of my elementary years. My teachers knew of my mother's mental illness and were always very compassionate towards her. One of my teachers, Miss Tassone, stated how impressed she was to see how completely dedicated they were to me and to my well-being. "Your parents are very concerned about you, more so than the average parent," she would say. Miss Tassone, who became a lifetime friend to me, also stated that if my parents didn't have the problems they had, she thinks they would have remained together. Despite their challenges, there seemed to exist a deep love and respect between them. All of these comments made me contemplate their struggles more deeply.

My dad and I always spent Halloween night together. One year, he drove me to the rich area by the lake to trick or treat because I convinced him that the candy was better there. Whatever car my dad had at the time, it was guaranteed to be in bad shape. He changed cars as often as he changed apartments. He would usually get evicted for not paying his rent, and his jalopies were always a step away from the junkyard. This car, however, was the nicest car he ever had, and I could tell he was proud of it.

After trick or treating, my dad and I were driving along a dark road. All of a sudden, my window began going up and down. I was scared and asked my dad why it was doing that. He said, "It's a Halloween ghost!" As the window kept going up and down, I became more fascinated and somewhat excited that there was a Halloween ghost in the car! Finally, he showed me that he had this crazy new thing called "electric windows" in his car and that he could control the windows from his side. We laughed and he especially thought that the whole experience was very funny.

My dad could have had a better quality of life, but he chose to not accept the disability pay from the military that he was entitled to. On some level, he felt if he accepted that money, then he was admitting he had a problem. So instead, he found random sign-painting jobs and lived without a steady income or insurance. Consequently, he struggled to make a living. He never owned a home, never had a 401K or a pension. He could not afford to even buy dentures, so he spent much of his adult life toothless. He never seemed to have enough to eat, and his clothes were usually bought at the thrift store.

My dad lived in a one-room apartment. His apartment was as meager as they come. He had an old chair that he surely found in someone's garbage. Throughout most of his life, he did not own a bed. He could not afford a mattress, so he made do with his creation of cinder blocks, a piece of plywood, and piece of foam rubber on top of that. He had the same routine every morning, which included eating his wheat germ and doing some exercises in his room. Despite his humble circumstances, he would often sit in his apartment in the evenings, writing poetry and plays or reading history books. He loved the theater, even though he could not afford to attend it. One year, he auditioned for a part in the local performance about Mary, Queen of Scots and was cast in a great role. I was so proud to be able to sit in the audience and watch him perform.

My dad knew many people in our community, including local attorneys and some of our councilmen. He set up boat rides for me on Lake Erie with some of his friends who had their own boats. He was friendly, kind, and outgoing with everyone, regardless of their backgrounds. He was very intelligent and well read, and he would get into great conversations with others. Surely, the people he was interacting with had no idea what simple circumstances he was living in.

One of my dad's friends, who was a city councilman, told me that my dad had tried for years to get a family convicted for injuring me as a baby. I had no recollection of this event and had never heard a thing about it until it was mentioned to me in passing. When my parents were still together, they had a lady friend in their apartment building who offered to watch me while they ran an errand. When they returned a short while later, they discovered that I had a very red backside that eventually turned black and blue. Later, the lady admitted that her "retarded" son had beaten me. According to this councilman, my dad was fiercely protective and was still approaching the city prosecutor, years later, trying to get him to press charges.

My dad carried many burdens that I was never fully aware of. He spent the holidays alone in his apartment without the home-cooked meals others were enjoying. Christmas and Thanksgiving were particularly difficult for him. I would see him for a few minutes in the evening on those days, and even though he would put on a happy face for me, I could tell his loneliness had gotten the best of him and that he had been crying.

As I grew older, I observed that my dad's circumstances seemed so unfair and so unfitting for such a wise, talented, and good person. Despite the harsh circumstances he faced in his life, he didn't complain. In fact, my dad would often say, "If you ask God for five things and He gives you one of those five things, then spend your life thanking Him for that one thing." He told me on several occasions that I was his "one thing."

My parents continued to work well together in spite of their struggles. I had many bouts of tonsillitis as a young child and with those came high fevers. Miraculously, my mom was always healthy enough to take care of me during these stressful times. She was frequently on the phone speaking to the doctors when the fevers would spike. On a number of occasions, my parents took me to the emergency room to get my fever down. I remember hating it when the hospital put me in ice baths. I would cry at the discomfort of the freezing water, and my parents were both there to comfort me. It seemed my mom's mothering instinct overpowered her illness during these times of crisis.

Other than the tonsillitis, I was a healthy kid. I was a very active girl in the neighborhood, and my friends and I would put on shows in my kitchen for our families. Even though Grandma wouldn't normally let him in the house, she made an exception for those nights of endless entertainment. It was a treat when my dad could sit in the kitchen and watch our performances.

As I grew older, my dad would blow the horn once in front of my house, which was his signal that he was there. I would meet him at the back door where he would bring me chewing gum. We would talk for a few minutes and share the happenings of the day. When it was really cold, he would stand in the back stairwell. We started a tradition of hiding a penny above the door jam.

Every time he came to visit, we would look to see if the penny was still there, and, of course, it was always there. It was our little secret.

Because of my mother's escalating illness, my dad was the one who usually attended my school events. He helped me make a kite for the kite-flying contest. He came to my track meets. He also taught me a song and dance routine, which I performed for my school class. On one occasion, I was asked to be the narrator for the school play. I was so excited when my parents and my grandma came to watch. To have all three of them there was a dream come true!

My mother's illness brought its share of collateral damage. I made a friend at school named Teresa, and we quickly became inseparable. I invited Teresa to spend the night at my house. It was the first and last sleepover that I ever hosted in elementary school. A few hours after we laughed ourselves to sleep, we woke up to my mom screaming and slamming the kitchen cupboard doors. Of course, Teresa was very frightened. The next thing we knew, my mom was on the phone telling Teresa's parents to come and pick up their daughter. There was no rhyme or reason for this behavior; it was just an impulsive thing she was doing because she was sick. My grandma was pleading with my mom to stop what she was doing and to let Teresa stay, but my mom kept going. She had a glazed look in her eyes and was very out of it. I cried hysterically and begged her to let Teresa stay. Eventually Teresa's mom showed up with a puzzled look on her face. She took Teresa home that night, and I buried my head in my pillow and cried. Soon after that, Teresa moved away, and we never saw or spoke to each other again.

CHAPTER 7

As I entered my junior high years, my mother's efforts to self-medicate increased. Unfortunately, our small home was within walking distance of six bars. I quickly became familiar with each bar since my grandma would send me to find my mom and bring her home. My mom's drinking was getting out of hand. She couldn't hold any type of job, and she stopped taking her medication completely.

One of the regulars I would see at the bars was a man people called "G-man." The *G* stood for "garbage" and referred to his previous career as a garbage man. He was considered the town drunk. One morning, I woke up and walked up the street to get my friend to play. In the yard next to mine,

I stumbled across G-man, laying in the lawn, all bloodied and unconscious. I ran home and told my grandma. She called the police, and the ambulance took him away; we later received word that he had died. Apparently, someone had beaten him badly. I didn't view this event as scary. In fact, I found it a bit interesting. However, looking back, this was a turning point for me in that I became much more protective of my mom. When I would go into a bar to retrieve her, I felt more anxious to get her out of there quickly. I soon realized that the bars could be dangerous places, especially for my ill mother.

As my mother's mental health continued to decline, my grandma sought help from our extended family. One evening, our relatives came to the house. They sat with Grandma and tried to talk my mom into admitting herself into a mental hospital. As the family spoke to my mom, they poured themselves drink after drink until their speech became slurred. Even as a young girl, I could tell this was not the best way to approach the situation. None of them were well equipped to deal with this mental illness, so they just did the best they could. There was no training or counseling provided for any of the family members. I watched my mom become more and more restless as they threw out many threatening statements with the hope of scaring her into admitting herself into a hospital. Listening to the whole conversation made me very anxious. When the relatives finally left, I was relieved.

A few moments after they drove away, Mom's agitation exploded and she lashed out at my grandma, who had been very calm and non-threatening during the entire night. As Grandma stood up and walked away from the kitchen table, my mom physically charged at her and began shaking her. I immediately threw myself between their two bodies and was attempting to hold my mother back. My mom's hand went over my shoulder and reached Grandma, who went crashing to the floor, landing on her hip. My mom looked shocked and confused and ran out of the house. Grandma instructed me to call the police, which I did immediately. The ambulance came and took Grandma to the emergency room and after some testing was completed, it was determined that her hip was broken. The police eventually found my mom in a bar. They brought her home to get a few things, then they admitted her into the mental hospital.

The following six weeks were very difficult indeed. Grandma spent that time in the hospital and in a rehabilitation center, and my mom stayed in a mental hospital. This left Uncle Wally and I alone, so Grandma arranged for an extended family member to stay at our house. I missed my grandma very much and did not want to sleep in the bedroom without her, so I put a blanket over the piano bench, making a mini tent in our living room, and slept that way for six weeks.

During this difficult period, the family member who was helping in the home happened to mention to me that I had been conceived "out of wedlock." Honestly, I barely knew what that meant, but I found it interesting, so I mentioned it to my dad when he came to visit that evening. When my dad heard this, he became irate. To begin with, there was no love lost between my dad and my mom's extended family. They never liked each other for many reasons. As I was telling this to my dad in front of my house, the family member who was staying at the home began backing Grandma's car out of our driveway to go somewhere. My dad saw this, and he stood at the side of the driveway and began screaming and swearing at them with his loud booming voice. This person who had revealed this revelation about my life to me continued to angrily back the car out of the driveway while covering her ears with one hand. It was safe to say that she and my dad hated each other.

During this very long six-week period, I would take the city bus to visit my mother in the mental hospital. On one particular visit, she looked at me and asked if I could please get her out of the hospital because there was a lady in her ward who thought she was a cat. Even though my mom seemed scared at the time, it was clear that she was getting better.

CHAPTER 8

It was one of the happiest days of my life when my grandma came home from the hospital. Eventually, my mom came home as well, and life seemed to return to normal.

Things settled down again and I eventually joined the German Club at my junior high school. The club was planning a trip to Germany for those who could afford it. I was so excited about the prospect of being able to travel somewhere that I was willing to do whatever I needed to do to make the money so I could go on the trip. I learned that the neighborhood paperboy had quit, so I asked my dad if I could take over the paper route. It was an early morning route, and I would be delivering papers in the dark and in some very questionable places. There was no hesitation on my dad's part when it came time to answer my question. He simply said, "ABSOLUTELY NOT!"

When I told my grandma what my dad's response was, she thought he was being unreasonable, and, in so many words, she gave me permission to take over the paper route. So without my dad's knowledge, I woke up early in the cold Cleveland mornings and delivered papers for most of the school year. It was a hard job, but I eventually made the money I needed to go to Germany. My grandma gave me one hundred dollars for spending money and off I went! It was a great trip. Being a little bit boy crazy at the time, I paid more attention to the boys on the trip than I did to the beautiful sites. The highlight of my trip was buying a cuckoo clock in the Black Forest. I brought the clock home and since neither Grandma nor I could figure out how to set it up, I placed it in the attic in a box with the hope that someone could help me assemble it.

One night, shortly after the Germany trip, I was watching TV and heard on the news that a girl in my area was kidnapped and murdered. She happened to be a papergirl. This story deeply disturbed me. Up until this time, I had never heard of someone killing a child. I didn't realize there were people in the world that would do something so awful. On some level, I realized that my dad had been right all along about not wanting me to do that paper route.

Life moved on and I made a new best friend in junior high named Barb. We had so much fun together. Barb's mother, Elaine, was one of the dearest women one could ever meet. She took my mother under her wing and would invite her over to her home. Sometimes the two moms would do things together, like go to lunch. In spite of my mom's odd behavior and inability to carry on a conversation, Elaine kept being a kind, compassionate friend. This made me so happy. I felt proud to see my mother doing normal mom things. It was an added bonus that Barb was my best friend. Sometimes we would laugh so hard that we would pee our pants.

Adolescence was rough and I became very shy in junior high school. For some reason, I had a tough time looking people in the eye when they spoke to me. When our family would go to extended family get-togethers, I always stayed close to my grandma.

As the junior high years moved on, I became increasingly aware of my grandma's heart problems. She had some minor heart attacks that were very scary. On occasion I would watch her make a concoction of onions that she would put on her chest with the hope to remedy the chest pain that she was having. Despite these problems and her increasing age, she still ran the house.

Grandma loved having parties with her friends. Since she didn't like to leave Uncle Wally and I alone for very long, she usually had Friday night poker nights at our house. They were so fun! When one of Grandma's friends got up to go to the bathroom, I was allowed to sit in their place and make decisions for their hand. Usually the person sitting next to me would give me tips on what to do. They had an open bar and on occasion I would get to mix drinks for them. They would direct me by saying, "Fill the cup with this," "Then add that," etc.

As much as I loved having my grandma's friends over, there was one friend I did not like. Her name was Anna. Anna was a mean old lady. When my grandma was hospitalized for a short time for a mild heart attack, Anna called the house and I answered the phone. Referring to my grandma's heart attack, Anna began yelling, "See what you did! See what you did!" I put down the phone, heartbroken, shocked, and confused. Had I somehow caused my grandma's heart attack? When my grandma came home from the hospital, I told her what Anna had said, and she became angry and upset. Anna didn't come to the house much after that.

~

Even though I was around a lot of drinking, I had no desire to drink as a teenager. The only exception was the time that I stole a bottle of gin from my grandma's liquor cabinet. I took it down to the basement and tried to get drunk, simply because I was curious what it felt like. I was only able to get one or two gulps down before I started gagging. I returned the bottle and never touched gin again. Since our family had a strong Swiss and German background, I was allowed to have some beer with the family while we ate Sunday dinner. That was the extent of my drinking career.

I developed a great interest in religion during my junior high years. I had been saying bedtime prayers since I was a little girl. I would recite a German prayer that my grandma taught me, still adding, "and please don't ever let Grandma, Mom, Dad, or Uncle Wally ever die." Additionally, my dad spent many hours teaching me about Jesus Christ. The first Christmas gift I remember receiving was a book entitled *Stories of*

Jesus that my dad said Santa left at his apartment for me. He was a devoutly religious and spiritual man who didn't believe in organized religion and who never attended church. Since none of my family attended church and my mom no longer went on Easter Sunday because of her illness, I decided to explore different religions. I went to my friends' churches, including catechism classes for both Catholic and Lutheran churches. I called the Baptist church and even though I knew no one there, I had their bus pick me up a few times to take me to their meetings. I walked to our little neighborhood Presbyterian church, and I ended up attending there most frequently. I asked a lot of questions and began really searching out what the differences were in the various churches' beliefs. I ended up finding a church that answered my questions. I was very happy and felt that I had found truth. My prayers became more meaningful and heartfelt. I would often put on my mother's old Carpenter's cassette tape and in place of a prayer, I would sing to God the song,

"We've Only Just Begun." I was even more excited about what I could do with my life, with Him by my side.

Chapter 9

As high school approached, I realized that it was time that I had my own room. There were only two bedrooms in our house, and Uncle Wally slept in the living room, so I decided to make a bedroom out of the hallway between the two upstairs bedrooms. This way, I was between my mom and my grandma.

One day I made a new friend named Leslie who was going to try out for cheerleading. I had planned on trying out for the cross-country team but then decided to follow my new ambitious friend. I was so nervous when tryouts came. We sat along the gym floor on numbers. One of the things we were being graded on was the loudness of our voices. Finally, they called my name.

My heart was pounding as I stood in front of the judge's table. I was asked to do a cartwheel, splits, round-off, etc. Next the judges asked me to shout my cheer. The gym was silent. Out came this extremely loud voice that surprised everyone, including myself. The judges were all laughing and smiling because I had been so much louder than any of the other girls that day. That night, I found out that I made the squad. I knew in a roundabout way that I had my mom to thank for this new opportunity. Even though I would never be able to sing as well as she used to sing, apparently her capacity for volume was passed onto me.

~

High school started and I was so excited to be a freshman! One morning I put on a little mascara before school and as I was walking out the door, my grandmother asked, "Why are you wearing that black stuff around your eyes?" I was a little embarrassed, but I quickly got over that feeling and continued to wear makeup. Grandma was a little old fashioned but soon accepted the fact that I was growing up.

Freshman year was moving along very well. I worked hard in school and was getting good grades. It was just a few weeks before Christmas, and that was always a magical time in our home. I was happy and excited about life. Everything seemed to be going very well.

One day my grandma started complaining of severe chest pain. After going to the doctor, it was determined that she had a heart attack, and she was admitted into the hospital. I walked to the hospital after school and entered the cardiac care unit. There was my grandma, lying in bed, yet still her same old self. Something felt very different this time, however, and it was clear that both she and I were feeling it. I developed a huge lump in my throat, and the only way I was able to stop myself from crying was to rapidly talk about what was going on at school. I shared with her lots of details about my latest boy crush. Visiting hours were over and it was time to go. I gave my grandma a hug, then I began walking out the door. As I headed towards the elevator, we looked at each other through the glass wall of her room for as long as we could. I walked down the hospital hall and without really knowing why, I cried as I walked home. I went to bed that night and slept in the bed that Grandma and I had shared all those years.

I woke up suddenly around 4 a.m. It was dark outside, yet I couldn't sleep. I walked downstairs to the living room and noticed that all the lights in the house were on. I called for my mother, but she was not in the house for some reason. Uncle Wally and I were alone in the house and he was asleep. I became very frightened. The phone suddenly rang—it was an extended family member.

"We'll be down there soon," they said.

"What do you mean? Why are you coming here in the middle of the night?" I asked.

"Grandma died. Did you not know that?"

68

I was stunned. I put the phone down, fell on the floor, and sobbed. My nightmare was coming true. My whole world was my grandma. I had never felt so much pain and agony than I did at that moment.

A few hours later, my mom resurfaced. I didn't know for sure where she had been. Her illness was getting so bad she rarely spoke to anyone. When morning came, I just sat in the kitchen by myself, feeling scared and in shock. My uncle showed up a few hours later. He came and took a few things from the house, including my grandmother's box of Buffalo nickels then quickly left. Clearly, he was worried my mom would not be able to take care of the valuable nickels, which, of course, was true. I looked at Uncle Wally and at my mom, who were both sitting lifelessly in the house. At that moment, I realized how alone I was in the world.

My grandmother's funeral was a very painful thing to go through. For a variety of reasons, I was scared of my mother's family, so I asked my high school counselor to go to the funeral with me. She kindly agreed. It was too upsetting to be there all alone. My mom cried during the funeral but didn't really talk to anyone. She was extremely detached from her surroundings. Her eyes were crazy looking, yet you could see she was feeling incredible pain.

Shortly after my grandma's death, my Uncle Wally was placed in a nursing home. I would ride the city bus to visit him, and he would just put his head down and cry. The nursing home just left him alone in his bed most of the time. His room was very cold and sterile. He often said that he wished he had been the one to die instead of his sister. He passed away shortly after Grandma died.

~

As the holiday season approached, I was overcome with despair. My mother, my dog, and I were now alone in the house. At fourteen years old, I felt as if life was over, and I didn't want to live any longer. I was in so much pain. All that hope and anticipation I had felt for life was now dead inside of me. As I sat looking out the window at the gray Cleveland sky, I began contemplating suicide. I just wanted to die so I could be with my grandma again. There was no point to living.

Suddenly, I heard this quiet but audible voice in my head, which said, "Turn on the radio." I dismissed the voice and again it said, "Turn on the radio." This time I listened. As I turned the radio on, to my surprise, the station had just started to play the Carpenters' song, "We've Only Just Begun." The song was perfectly starting at the beginning, and I hadn't missed a note of the song. Now this was the 1980s, and that song was already past its time and was rarely played. I was immediately overcome with an amazingly feeling of comfort and love, and I felt this warmth go through my entire body. I had never felt such a powerful feeling like that before. It was clear to me that God was sending me a message. This time He was singing this song to me. That experience strengthened me and even though I felt great despair and sadness, I was able to start to feel a sense of hope again.

It was a week before Christmas, and there were no decorations in the house. It didn't feel anything like the Christmases of the past. Grandma was not in the kitchen baking her Christmas cookies. I remembered how I would help Grandma with the holiday baking. "If she hadn't died, I would be standing here, putting my thumb in the middle of the cookies and filling them with jelly," I thought. As I continued to watch the gray Cleveland weather outside the front room window, I saw a station wagon pull up. Tied to the top of the car was a big Christmas tree. It was Mr. Lee, a man from my church. I watched him as he untied the tree and then carried it up to our front door where I was waiting for him. He came in and helped me put the tree in the stand. I thanked him and he left. I ran and got the box from the attic with all the Christmas tree lights and ornaments, and then I decorated the tree. That night, the tree lit up the house and became a symbol of hope for me.

My mother was too ill to cook, so at fourteen years old, I began the routine of walking to the neighborhood grocery store and with the limited money we had, I picked out food that I could make. It was tough going for a while. I invited two people over for dinner one night and tried to make a homemade pizza. The crust was hard as a rock and completely inedible. The guests smiled and scraped the pizza toppings off onto their plate and put the crust to the side. I soon learned to make several different things for dinner, but no food would ever taste as good as my grandma's food.

It was almost Christmas Eve and as Cleveland weather would have it, it brought with it some snow. There were no gifts under the tree that year. It was a very different kind of Christmas.

I decided I had to make a choice. I could sit at home and do nothing, or I could do something productive, so I went to the kitchen and tried my hand at baking cookies. They didn't turn out very well. Nevertheless, I decided that I would deliver them to my friends on that cold snowy night. I put on my long underwear, my red footie pajamas, my snow boots, hat, gloves, and a scarf. I tied a small sheet around my neck and mouth so I would look something like Santa Claus, then I headed out to deliver my cookies. It was a fourteen-year-old girl versus the elements. I walked three miles in the snow to my friend's house and delivered my first batch of cookies. I kept going house to house until I had delivered all five batches of the cookies. When I was done, I walked home in the freezing weather.

As I walked through the dreary town, I felt myself get stronger and stronger. The fiercer the wind became, the more I pushed against it. The more snow that fell, the quicker and harder I trudged through it. Although there were no gifts that year at my house, I felt like I had been given a great gift that night. I found a renewed energy and determination to handle my new world alone without my grandmother.

CHAPTER 10

Spring breathed new life into our little home on Magee Street, and I began doing the traditional Saturday yard work. Even though I felt sad because this was something that Grandma and I used to do together, there was also a feeling of comfort in this chore because I knew that cleaning up the yard was something that would have made her happy. I did my best to keep the weeds and hedges under control, but unfortunately, the yard deteriorated compared to what it had looked like.

I even tried my hand at canning food. I found a big Mason jar that Grandma had used, and I filled it with tomatoes, put it in boiling water until the seal popped, and then put it in the cellar. I also found a deal on a bunch of fresh green beans, so I froze them and put them in the deep freezer in the basement. I never actually ate the beans or the tomatoes, but it felt good having some food in the basement in case the cupboards went completely bare.

My mother continued to be very sick and was not able to work most of the time. Meanwhile, I rode the city bus to and from school each day. I would wait for the bus at the end of my street. One of the younger teachers from my school lived nearby and met at the bus stop one day and asked if I would like a ride. I happily jumped in his warm car to avoid riding the cold and dirty bus. One day, he asked if I would like to go to Florida with him for spring break. This was such an odd thing to say. Afterall, he was a teacher that I looked up to and a popular and well-liked coach in our high school. I became uncomfortable and told him that I needed to take care of my mother. I didn't accept his rides to school after that.

I always felt a level of anxiety when I would come home from school. If my mother wasn't in our house, then I knew she was out drinking. I would put my backpack down on the couch, and then I'd head out and begin the walk to look for her. I went bar to bar until I found her. I was always appalled at how frequently there seemed to be some weird guy sitting next to my mom, trying to hit on her even though she couldn't carry on a conversation because of her illness. It was also evident from her physical appearance that she was a very sick woman.

One man in particular named Russ seemed to be hanging around her quite a bit. While I was retrieving my mother from a bar one day, Russ stopped me and said in a slurred voice, "I love your mother." I became very irritated with him and reminded him that because of her illness she wasn't able to talk to him, so he couldn't love her because he didn't even know her. Surely Russ had plenty of issues himself, but because he was so much more functional than my mom, to me he was a scumbag drunk. I didn't want him near my mother. I didn't trust him.

After walking in the door from school a few days later, I got the shock of a lifetime. There were Scumbag Russ's shoes sitting by the door, and I saw him on the living room couch trying to take advantage of my sweet mother. I was a pretty quiet and even-keeled kid who rarely got mad, but at that moment I suddenly felt the strength of ten men. Scumbag Russ scrambled to his feet as I yelled, "Get the hell out of here!" I took his shoes and threw them out the front door onto the steps and sidewalk below. He kept saying in a slurred voice, "but I love her," and I just kept yelling back, "Get the hell out of here!" As I was getting ready to grab him and physically remove him from our home, he ran out of the house, and I slammed the door behind him.

I scolded my mother and yelled at her, "What were you thinking?" After hearing my own words, I stopped myself. What was I saying? My mom didn't know what she was thinking. She was mentally ill. She was an incapacitated child who had a dazed look and was detached from reality. Trying to reason with her was a waste of time. My heart softened and I felt sorrow for my mother and the horrible illness that robbed her of the ability to reason and make decisions. After that event, Russ never showed his face again at our house, and I never saw him at the bars or around my mother.

Now that I was fifteen years old, I decided it was time for me to get a real job. I was very busy with school and extracurricular activities, but we needed more money. I got a job at Burger King, the very place my mother was fired from years earlier. On the weekends I would close, which meant I wouldn't get home until 3:30 in the morning. Those were tough shifts, but I did the best I could. I was often so tired from work, school, and other activities that during my work breaks, I would go into the single stall bathroom and lay on the greasy floor with the hope of catching a nap for a few minutes. Those naps were the only way I could make it through the night.

I didn't like it when the supervisor at work yelled at me for something that I didn't do correctly. One time I was reprimanded for not getting the burgers out quickly enough. After being mildly scolded, I felt a lump building up in my throat, so I took a break, went to the bathroom, and cried. Even though the criticism was justified, I just didn't have the strength to handle anyone yelling at me on top of everything else I was dealing with.

It was getting difficult for me to hold it all together, but I pressed on. I began losing weight. When the next round of cheerleading tryouts was over, my coach called me and said that I had made the squad for the next year *with the condition* that I would have to gain some weight. I hung up the phone and felt hurt. Even though I was certain she knew that my mother was ill, the coach never asked me about my home situation, nor did she ever offer to bring over a meal. I'm assuming that she didn't know that my mom and I didn't have a lot of food to begin with and that it was my responsibility to buy and make any food we ate. I felt very misunderstood and alone and unsure how to ask for help.

My guidance counselor eventually moved and changed jobs, and the school offered no help with my situation. At times it actually added to the problem. One morning I woke up and realized that I literally did not have one clean thing to wear, so I quickly did some laundry, threw my clothes on, and raced to school.

When I walked into the attendance office, the attendance lady asked me, "Why are you late?"

I replied, "I didn't have any clean clothes, so I had to do some laundry."

The attendance lady proceeded to make an angry face at me and yelled, "You are so irresponsible!" I walked away, and once again went into the restroom and cried.

I went home from school that day and opened the front door of the house expecting to see Cocoa.

However, that day there was no Cocoa. I looked and looked and couldn't find him anywhere. My heart sank. I couldn't handle another loss. I made phone calls, and no one knew where he was. Cocoa was getting old and it was a lot of work to take care of him, but the loss of my dog that day brought back all the pain of losing my grandmother. I further grieved the happy home that I once knew.

Shortly after the disappearance of my dog, I learned that my extended family was going to sell my grandma's house and that my mother and I needed to find an apartment. This was devastating news. I loved my home. All of my memories of my grandma, Uncle Wally, and my dog were in that home. That home was a great sense of security for me. I felt sick inside.

While getting ready for the move, I was going through some papers one afternoon and stumbled across the letter that I had written years earlier about "The Most Wonderful Woman in the World." It was the letter in which I requested the TV show to send my grandmother to Switzerland. The letter was folded and tucked away into some of her personal things. It was clear that Grandma had intercepted the letter and had put it in a safe place where she could treasure it.

The home sold fairly quickly. My mom and I found an old apartment in a building on the other side of town. I cried and cried when we had to leave her home. It was as if my grandma had died all over again.

CHAPTER 11

Hate is a strong word, but I *hated* our new apartment. It was a one-bedroom unit on the third floor. The windows would get thick ice on the inside in the winter, and my mom and I would sweat to death in the summer. Mom slept on the couch and I slept in the one and only bedroom. One of the rules I established early on is that there would be no smoking in the apartment. I did not want to smell like cigarette smoke and with such a small space, I definitely didn't want to be suffocating on my mother's cigarette smoke. Nevertheless, on occasion I would come home from school and find the entire apartment filled with smoke. Regardless of the temperature, I would open all the windows and leave them open until the air cleared. This became a big source of frustration for me.

My routine of seeing my dad on a daily basis continued into my high school years. He would show up around 8:00 at night, and he would always bring me gum. We would talk or go for a ride in his car. He went through several cars and they were always on their last leg, yet he was always happy to have transportation.

One of the cars he owned was particularly memorable. The doors had the problem of falling off the hinges when someone opened them, so my dad tied a rope that went through the windows and around the roof so the doors would not fall completely off when someone got in and out of the car. Consequently, you could never roll the windows up all the way, and the car would get very cold inside. The car was so rusted out that there was a hole in the floor. I would watch the pavement of the street below when we were driving. My dad established an emergency procedure in case the floor fell out of the car. While pointing to a small vinyl strap over the passenger side mirror he would say, "Nan, grab onto this if the whole floor goes." Thankfully, I never had to use it because the strap could barely hold itself to the car, let alone hold the weight of a teenage girl.

One evening, I asked my dad to take me for a ride in his car so I could drive by the house of the boy whom I had a crush on. I just wanted to go by his house one time to see where he lived. I was fully expecting to fulfill my curiosity by simply driving by this boy's house, and that would be that. As we approached the house in my dad's loud jalopy, panic overcame me as I saw the boy outside mowing his lawn. Not only did I not want him to think I was stalking him, I certainly didn't want him to see me in the tin can on wheels, so I quickly ducked down on the floorboard and hoped the floor would not fall out in front of his house. My dad, seeing the humor in the situation, exclaimed, "I'm going to blow the horn! Should I blow it now? How about now?" We passed the house without incident, thankfully, and we laughed over that moment for quite some time.

High school was going well. I had good friends at church and at school, and I liked my classes. Even though I had an unusual home situation, I somehow maintained the dangerous naivety of a fifteen-year-old girl.

One day, my history teacher approached me and asked if I would like to be the representative of the high school and attend an all-expenses paid workshop in Washington, D.C. I was so excited that I immediately accepted his offer!

I attended the workshop and had a great time. Flying there and back alone on an airplane was very exciting. On my flight home, I sat next to a man named Carlzo. He was in his forties. He initiated a conversation by saying that he noticed I was reading some religious material. He went on to say how he had been trying to find God again in his life but was struggling to do so. I shared with him some facts about my life, including my mother's illness. He continued to speak for a while, and as the plane began to descend, he asked for my phone number with the hope that we could continue our conversation. I agreed and gave him my number. After all, he was a man trying to find God, and he was asking me for help. How could I not help him?

As we walked off the plane together, my dad quickly approached us, and he appeared very distressed. He began pointing to Carlzo while asking me, "Who is that? Were you talking to him?" I just dismissed his questions as hidden prejudice since the man was black. After all, my dad was an old Clevelander, and he didn't understand people as well as I did.

A few days later, Carlzo called me. He asked if he could pick me up so we could continue talking about God. Of course, I agreed. I always had a strong belief in God and was happy to share that belief with others. He pulled up in a Mercedes in front of my old apartment and having not told anyone where I was going, I climbed into his car and the two of us left together. Initially, I felt safe.

It was early in the day and I was anxious to help this poor man. After a few minutes of driving, he began playing suggestive music and singing the lyrics out loud. While looking at me, he sang something like, "Baby, tonight is our night." I immediately became uncomfortable. What had I gotten myself into?

After driving a little while, we pulled into a Cleveland ghetto, and he told me to stay in the car. He walked over to a young man and handed him a mysterious small bag. The young man handed him money in return, and Carlzo got back into the car. Now I knew I was in trouble, and I began praying for help. This man did not want to talk about religion or anything of the sort. He was looking at me like a piece of meat. We stopped at KFC and he bought me a meal. I should have run for help at that point, but for some reason I was too afraid. Thankfully, he drove me back to my apartment, and I couldn't get out of his car quickly enough. Unfortunately, Carlzo also got out of the car and asked if he could come upstairs to my apartment for a while. I said, "No, that's not a good idea. My mom isn't home." He kept pressuring me and I became more scared as we stood in front of my apartment.

Now for the past fifteen years of my life, I always saw my dad late in the evening, except for Sundays when we would visit my paternal grandparents earlier in the day. It was about 4:00 in the afternoon when I suddenly saw a flash of rust in front of me. It was my dad. He was driving his car much faster than it was surely capable of going. He made a very hurried U-turn in front of us. I barely got the words out of my mouth, "Oh, there's my dad," when Carlzo began running to his Mercedes. My dad jumped out of his car and began sprinting after the frightened man as he sped away in his car. The best way to explain my dad at that moment was pure rage. This big redheaded Scottish man—who his friends had described as "a nasty bar fighter" back in his drinking days—was let out of his cage. I'm certain that if my dad had caught Carlzo that day, he would have, at the very least, beaten him badly.

After the car sped away from him, my dad ran over to me yelling, "What is he doing here? What is that guy from the airport doing here?"

I just put my head in my hands and cried and said, "How did you know to come here, Dad?"

He replied with a softer voice, "I was working and just kept having this thought that said, 'Go check on Nancy, go check on Nancy,' so that's what I did."

A little while later, I received a call from a federal agent of some sort, stating they were investigating Carlzo and wanted to know what I knew about him. He proceeded to tell me that Carlzo had been in prison. I answered his questions and hung up the phone, sick to my stomach.

Chapter 12

A few months later, my sixteenth birthday finally arrived! I was so excited! I knew that driving a car wasn't in the works for me; in fact, I didn't even think about that. My mom and I would never have a car and my dad would not let me drive his safety hazard of a vehicle. I was excited because I could date! I told myself that I wouldn't date any boys until I was sixteen because I believed that was the right thing to do, so I had been waiting for this big day for a long time.

My latest crush was Eric, and unfortunately, his dad taught driver's ed at the high school. I was horrified to find out that of all the driver's ed teachers I could have been assigned to, I was given Eric's dad! I didn't have any driving experience at all, so I was very nervous how this was going to work.

With much trepidation, I began driver's education class. Thankfully, it was going well until it was time to drive on the freeway. It was my turn to drive, and there were two other students in the back seat. We were driving on a very busy freeway section by the airport. I was in the far outside lane, and Eric's dad instructed me to switch to the very inside lane. He repeated his instruction several times. Unfortunately, I didn't know how to make my way through all that traffic to be able to make that lane change. I became very nervous, thinking that my instructor was going to go home and tell Eric what a horrible driver I was. After being told once again to get to the inside lane, I suddenly panicked and made a hardleft turn. Our car quickly flew across many lanes of traffic. Horns were beeping all around us, and cars were dodging our car. Everyone screamed, including Eric's dad as he yelled, "You have just failed driver's ed!" Thankfully, we didn't crash into anyone and we didn't die that day, but I was mostly upset because I knew my chances with Eric had been ruined.

In spite of my big birthday finally arriving, there was a sense of sadness on that day. The holidays and birthdays that used to be filled with excitement were now filled with a sense of loss. Somewhere around my birthday, I came home from school and to my surprise, my mother handed me a box. I hadn't received a gift from my mother in years. She had been too sick to be able to shop and because of her illness, she rarely spoke. I opened the box and saw a knit hat and matching mittens. The knit hat had a big green plastic monster on the front. This was a hat and glove set for a young boy and perhaps the very last thing that a sixteen-year-old girl would ever be caught wearing.

I looked at the gift and laughed. It was funny. Then I cried. It struck me that this was an amazing feat that my mother had accomplished. It became clear to me that my mom had gotten on the city bus that day by herself, went to the mall, paid for the gift with the little money we had, and then came home. How difficult that must have been for her to do. The very act of her riding the bus alone in her current condition made me nervous. When we would ride the bus together, she would start laughing out loud, sometimes to the point where tears would run down her face. Other times, she would yell and argue with an imaginary person who wasn't there. What had she done that day on the bus when I wasn't there to help her? What a tender and meaningful act of love this was.

I also felt a wave of sadness wash over me because I realized that the hat was also a symbol of the illness that my mother suffered. There were no more gifts for holidays, no more baby dolls, and no more birthday parties. The best she could do was a little boy's knit hat with a plastic monster on it for a sixteen-year-old girl. The reality was raw and right in front of me. Overshadowing my sadness, however, was the great love and appreciation that I felt for my sweet mother in that moment.

My sixteenth birthday came and went and so did the boy that I had a crush on. I found out that he started dating a girl and they were now a couple, so there went that idea. Instead, my good friend threw a sixteenth birthday dinner date party for me. It was going to be my first date. However, the boy she set me up with never showed up. There was one moment when she was counting the couples at the table, and she said, "Two, four, six," and after a long pause, ". . . seven." It was a funny moment that we all laughed about it for years.

I had two very close girl friends who were sisters in another town, and I often rode my bike to their house to hang out for the night. I went to a church camp with one of the sisters, and we bunked together. We decided we weren't going to follow the schedule the leaders had put together for us. We just wanted to canoe and have fun. Long story short, even though neither of us were normally rebellious girls, we were both kicked out of the camp. Her dad, who was the minister of our congregation, picked us up in their family st-tion wagon and drove us home.

Despite our act of rebellion, their family let me stay at their house for several nights where I slept on the floor between the two sisters' beds. I remember watching how easily they could fall asleep, and it made me wonder why I couldn't fall into a deep sleep that easily. It ended up being one of the most fun summers I ever had. Even though they had a large family, they graciously fed me and let me stay at their house.

I had another close friend, Mark, who was a boy from my high school. He and his family were very kind to me. On occasion, they would take me out to eat, which I greatly appreciated. One evening, Mark and I walked into my apartment. Lo and behold, there was my mother, sitting on the couch in the dark, in her bra and underwear, smoking a cigarette. Without skipping a beat, she said "Hi, Mark!" as if it were perfectly normal to be sitting there in her bra and panties in front of a couple of teenagers. My mom also had restless leg syndrome, so she sat with her legs crossed while swinging her leg wildly around. I quickly helped her put her clothes on and once again asked her to please not smoke in the apartment. Mark handled the situation very well. Because we both knew that my mom was ill, we found humor in what we were seeing. We both laughed as if we were laughing at the follies of an innocent child.

During this time, my mom was hospitalized on a few occasions. My dear friend, Mike, would drive me to visit my mother in the hospital. I always appreciated how very sweet he was with both of my parents. They both sensed his goodness and they loved him. He would also take my mom and I out for ice cream. I felt very grateful for the kind and understanding friend he was. Mike was an amazing student and athlete and was given a full-ride scholarship to play quarterback at a top college. To my shock, he eventually went into a catatonic state one day and was also diagnosed with schizophrenia. It was a sudden onset and was so shocking. I couldn't wrap my mind around the fact that yet another important person in my life had been taken from me. His bright and extremely promising future had been torn from him as well.

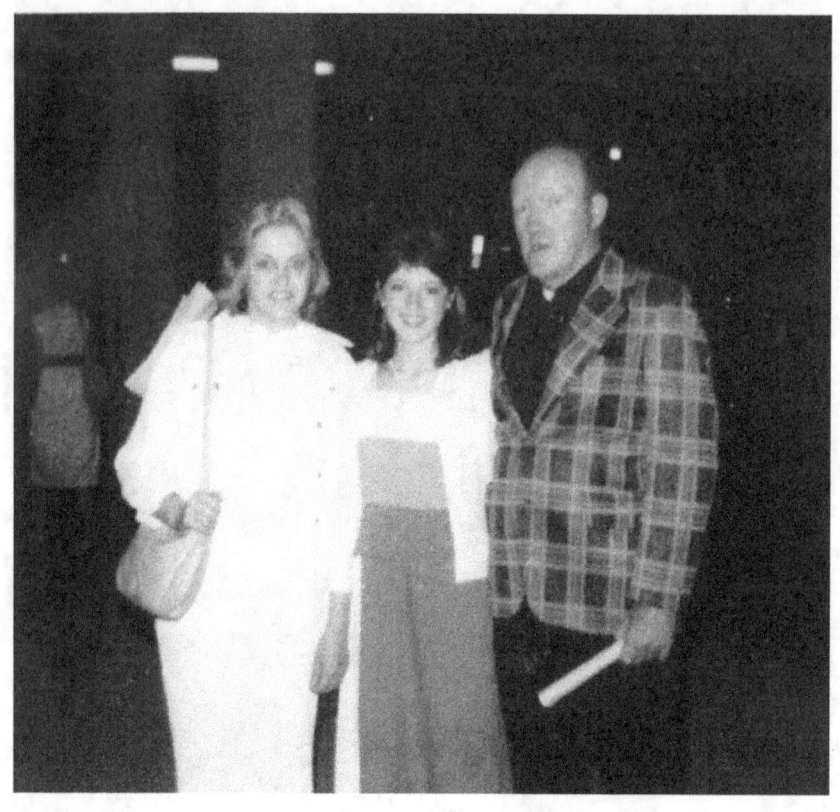

Nancy with her parents at high school graduation.

Chapter 13

I babysat a lot on the weekends. One summer day, I was asked to go on a trip with a family out of state so I could watch their two boys while they handled some business. They took me on a tour of the college they had attended, and I immediately fell in love with the campus. It was nestled in the mountains, and the environment was so beautiful and full of energy. I knew that was the place where I wanted to go to school one day. I visited their nursing school and gathered all the information I could. From that moment on, I became very focused on my goal to one day attend that university.

When I returned to Cleveland, I picked right back up with my teenage life. A few months later, I was walking on the city street to high school and noticed a boy who also walked to school. We seemed to be walking at the same time every day. I began seeing him more frequently, and we began to talk. He said his name was Dave, and we only lived a few blocks from each other. Soon after that, he became my first official boyfriend.

Dave and I had a lot of fun together. He came from a single-parent household, and his mother was also on welfare, so we had a lot in common. His mother had a car, and once in a blue moon we were allowed to drive it, but mostly we walked everywhere. We walked down to the valley and had picnics and rode bikes. I would go to his baseball games in the summer to cheer him on.

We frequently hung out at a young family's home that I knew from church. The family soon unofficially adopted us. We attended many events with them, ate many meals with them, and just had a lot of fun being at their house. They kept us healthy by feeding us lots of vegetables and good-quality protein, which neither of us had at home. We spent many nights going on ice cream runs with them as well. They were truly such great blessings to both of us.

One Friday evening, I spent the night at my girlfriends' house. To my chagrin, I came home the next morning and found a man's wallet in our apartment. I opened the wallet and discovered the man's address on his driver's license. Dave borrowed his mother's car and drove me to the man's house. He waited in the car as I walked up to the door and rang the bell. The owner of the wallet came to the door. He was a young guy who looked very hungover. I threw the wallet at him and proceeded to scold him for trying to take advantage of my mentally ill mother. He became visibly scared and reassured me that my mom had just let him spend the night at the apartment because he was too drunk to drive himself home. I could tell he was telling the truth, yet I continued to make my point clear that I was never to see him near my mother again. He was very apologetic. Dave and I drove away, and I never saw that man again.

~

One evening my mother and I were in our apartment. She spent most of her time asleep on the couch or if she was awake, she was simply too ill to carry on a conversation. Imagine my surprise, when she shot up from her laying down position and asked, "Nancy, have you had sex yet?"

When I heard that random and awkward question, I laughed out loud. It actually made me very happy to hear my mom ask me any question, even if it was this one! I told her the truth and said, "No, Mom. I'm going to wait until I get married to do that."

My mom replied, "Oh," and immediately laid back down and fell into a deep sleep on the couch. That was the closest thing to a conversa tion my mom and I had during my high school years.

My senior year of high school was coming up, and I decided to quit some of my extracurricular activities. This went against all the normal paths that everyone else seemed to be following, but I really didn't care. I needed to get another job in addition to my usual babysitting jobs, and I needed to save money to go to college. I also wanted to spend as much time as I could with my parents during that last year.

Dave and I ended up getting jobs together at the Beef Coral. The Beef Coral was a few steps below your typical fast-food place. The place was dirty, but it brought in a paycheck for us, so we did what we needed to do. We also worked odd jobs together for that entire school year and saved money so that we would have the funds to go to the prom. One of our high school teachers hired us to rake the acorns in her yard. We stashed our money away and we were very frugal.

I spent many nights that year doing the usual thing of pulling my mom out of bars. I was continually amazed to find some strange guy trying to hit on my obviously sick mother. I had no fear when it came to confronting these guys. Sometimes there would be an argument, but luckily, they always backed down and I usually left with the last word. It was very stressful and honestly exhausting to always be worried about where my mom was, all the while trying to be a normal teenage girl.

It was soon prom time. Dave picked me up and my mom came down to the front of the apartment to watch the two of us leave. She didn't say anything; she just stood there and looked at us and gazed into outer space. We drove over to our adopted family's home, and they took some pictures and saw us off.

Graduation day finally arrived. My friend Lisa surprised me and bought me a cute three-piece dress. Somehow, she knew that I didn't have anything nice to wear to graduation. After I walked across the stage and received my diploma, all the families met in the gym. I looked around and it seemed that all the girls were crying except for me. In many ways, I had already moved on from high school. I was ready to get on with the rest of my life. I was excited for my future.

I spent the summer working three jobs and saving my money. My dad bought me a bike, and I rode it to all of my places of work. One morning I locked my bike outside the restaurant I was cleaning. When I came out, my bike was gone. Someone had stolen it. It was probably the cheapest ten-speed bike you could buy, but it was my only method of transportation. I was devastated. I eventually found an old broken bike and made do with that.

As the end of the summer approached, I realized that despite my very best budgeting efforts, I was short a few hundred dollars for my upcoming college expenses. I became discouraged. I had worked myself almost to death at my three jobs and had saved all my money for college. I wasn't sure how or why I was coming up short.

One evening I was working at the milkshake station at the Beef Corral restaurant and began to feel very discouraged about my financial situation. I took a break and went to the bathroom and knelt on the floor and prayed. I cried and poured out my heart and asked God to help me figure out how to make things work financially. I had no idea how to come up with that last two hundred dollars that I needed for college, and I hadn't even added in any money for new clothes and shoes, which I desperately needed. I got off my knees and with my head hanging low, I went back to work.

Within minutes of returning to work at the milkshake station, Mrs. Gregg walked into the restaurant. Mrs. Gregg was a very nice lady from my church. She was a large woman who was fairly loud. She hurried up to the counter and said, "Nancy, did you hear?" I had no idea what she was talking about. Mrs. Gregg went on to say that she was at the church that day, and a women's organization happened to call the church office while she was there. They said they were trying to contact me because I was chosen to be the recipient of their $250 scholarship! They were unable to get a hold of me because our home phone had been disconnected due to nonpayment. Mrs. Gregg went on to say that they were so impressed with my application that they were doubling the amount of the award to $500! I had forgotten that I had applied for that scholarship a few months earlier.

As soon as Mrs. Gregg finished speaking, I felt an amazing feeling of love sweep through my body. It was that same feeling of love that I had felt when I was fourteen and was told to turn on the radio. Because of this surprise scholarship, not only would I be able to meet my schooling obligations that year, but I would also be able to buy some clothes and new shoes. That evening I tried not to cry happy tears into the customer's milkshakes.

CHAPTER 14

The most exciting and the most dreaded day finally arrived. It came time to leave for college. This was an exhilarating yet very painful time for me. I was filled with guilt and worry when I thought about leaving my mother. My grandmother's words which she had spoken to me when I was a young girl kept running through my head, "One day you will go to college, and when you do, you should go to college in a different state. Do not stay here and go to school." My decision may not have been the right decision for everyone in my situation, but I knew it was the right course for me. Somehow, I knew that I would never have a life of my own if I stayed in Cleveland. I also knew that if my mother had been well, she would have wanted me to leave so that I could have my own adventure.

It was time to put a plan in place so that my mom could be looked after. In addition to the help from some agencies that were checking on her, she had extended family members who took her out to eat on occasion. I relied mostly on my dad, however, who said that he would check on her every day, and he did just that.

I knew that it was going to be painful for my parents when I left for college. My dad stated that he built his whole world around me, and now he was asking himself what he would do with his life. My parents took me to the airport as I left for my freshman year. My mom was detached and sullen. The only words she spoke at the airport were, "I hate this day."

After I left, my dad did a great job of taking care of my mom. He brought her food on a regular basis. To be sure she had a good meal, he would take her out to eat at the local restaurants. Since neither of them had a working telephone, he would pick her up twice a week, and the two of them would go to a pay phone and call me at college. My dad would put my mom on the phone, and often she would say nothing or something completely nonsensical, yet it was always comforting to know that she was there.

My freshman year was my very best year at school. I had so much fun and learned so many things. I met people from all over the world, and I worked hard at my studies.

I came home at Christmas and in the summer so I could work and make money. I always loved coming home and I loved seeing my parents. During one of my breaks, I wrote the following in my journal:

Saturday, January 3

I had the greatest experience with my mother. I've never ever really been able to talk to mom but last night she laid on one end of the couch and [I laid] on the other and I do believe her illness was lifted from her for that period as a gift for me. All of a sudden, we started talking about her high school days and how we were alike. She didn't like to drink a lot even though the family did. It was really like mother and daughter. She asked me really thought-through questions and really listened. I almost cried as we talked. It was a once in a lifetime experience for me and one I will never forget. She told me that after I was born my Dad said, "let's have a boy next." Then Mom said to me, "But we never did." My Mom is the greatest. I sensed her spirit and felt closer to her on this break than any other time in my life. I saw her as an individual more than ever. We're alike in many ways but we also have our differences. I feel like Mom and Dad feel secure in their lives because they have me. When I'm with them, I feel this coming from them. We all need someone to be strong in our lives. I'm so happy to be theirs.

. . .

Mom woke up as schizophrenic as ever. She rambled on to me about all kinds of nonsensical things—really far-out thoughts. It was so evident that she has a chemical imbalance. I felt so bad for her when she said, "I felt good last night but they did it to me again!" Poor poor thing. She was inside this little shell trying to make it work for her, trying to get out.

During the following year at college, I was able to save up some money from the job I had at a gas station and bring my mother out during the semester. I wanted her to see where I was going to school. I knew this was going to be an undertaking, but I missed my mom and I thought that maybe a trip could be good for her. I was living in a student apartment at the time with roommates. I wrote the following in my journal:

Friday, April 4

I've been feeling sick since Mom got here. My stomach was doing things all the way up to the airport. One reason I've been feeling so stressed out is because Mom will not do anything with me. She insists on staying in this apartment and lying on the couch all day. I came home today, and she had the apartment full of smoke. She's so depressed all the time. I feel like I shouldn't have brought her here and that it didn't make a difference. I hope she can snap out of it. It's so hard to reason with mental illness. My microbiology lab teacher is a doctor and he told me that after every attack/spell/delu-

sion of schizophrenia, brain damage occurs. Shane at work told me, "She does look like a crazy person . . . you can tell in her eyes." That hurts a little to think of my mother as a "crazy person." I know her to be so much more than that.

Sunday, April 6

Boy has this been a rough week. Mom is here and that is a sentence in itself. She's doing very very poorly. I'm feeling pretty down. This week she didn't want to do anything but lay on the couch and smoke cigarettes outside. I had so many things planned. I hoped this trip would be therapeutic for her. All she does is either look so depressed and not say anything or she laughs hysterically to herself. I'm so disappointed. Yesterday I took her to work out. I thought a little exercise would be good for her (the exercise bike, racquetball, etc.). While checking the clothes out, she had a swearing/anger spell in front of the girl at the counter. The girl took it personally and I tried to cover for Mom and I later explained the situation [to the girl]. I came home to a smoky apartment the day before that. This morning we all woke up to a rotten-egg-awful-burning smell. Mom had put two *eggs on to boil and went back to bed. My roommates are pretty upset and feel it was foolish for me to bring her here. Today I took her up in the mountains for a picnic. I kept saying, "Mom look at these beautiful mountains," but she kept looking straight ahead. She ate her food and laughed hysterically (to herself). I hurt because I'm realizing just how limited I am in helping her.*

My mom eventually went back to Cleveland, and I returned to my schooling.

CHAPTER 15

A few years passed and when I was still in college, my dad went to check on my mom and found her doubled up in pain. My dad took her to the city hospital where they admitted her. Although my mom had been in the mental hospital before, she had never been in the mainstream hospital, and it was clear that she was going to be very scared.

I miraculously found a way home. My friend gave me the money for an airline ticket, and I quickly boarded a plane and went to Cleveland.

When I walked into my mother's hospital room, I could see that she was visibly agitated, angry, and scared. The doctor announced they were going to do a liver biopsy. I stood next to my mom and held her hand while they put the needle in her abdomen. Her agitation could no longer be contained, and she turned to me and started yelling all kinds of things. "Why are you letting this happen to me?" She yelled and swore at me. Somehow in my mom's mind, all of her pain was my fault. Feeling bad for me, the doctor said, "Your daughter is trying to help you, Carol."

After several tests, the doctors discovered that my mother was in the final stage of cancer. The source of the cancer was unknown, but after doing a mammogram, breast cancer was ruled out. The doctors felt the cancer most likely originated in the lungs from smoking. They told me that she had only a few weeks to live.

My mom stayed in the hospital, but she was moved to the psychiatric floor. She quickly declined and it became apparent that she had only a few days, not weeks, to live.

I sat next to my mom's bed in her quiet room. My mom hadn't spoken much since her liver biopsy. They kept her on a morphine drip to help her stay comfortable, and this made her even sleepier and more detached than she usually was.

All of a sudden, my mother opened her eyes and looked at me with amazing clarity. She said, "Honey, you are all I have in this world." Then she simply closed her eyes and fell back into a deep sleep. Hearing those rare, beautiful, and clear words from my mother caused big tears to roll down my cheeks. I sat there for a few moments in her quiet room before a relative walked in and sat down next to me. A few moments later, my mom took one deep and final breath and she was gone.

I will never forget what happened next. Immediately, my entire body was filled with a distinct feeling that I had never felt before. It was a powerful love that was coming from outside my body into my body, and it was illuminating my whole being. For that short moment, I felt as if there was lovely warm water flowing through my veins, and then suddenly the feeling was gone. I knew that my mother and I had a brief window together in that room, a few seconds when she was no longer a prisoner of the violent thief that had stolen her life and ravaged her body for years. Her love could not be constrained. I withdrew to the corner of the room and broke down and cried.

My sweet and wonderful mother was gone. She was now free from the body that held her captive for so many years. She was now free to be her kind and wonderful self. Her suffering was over, and she had been taken home.

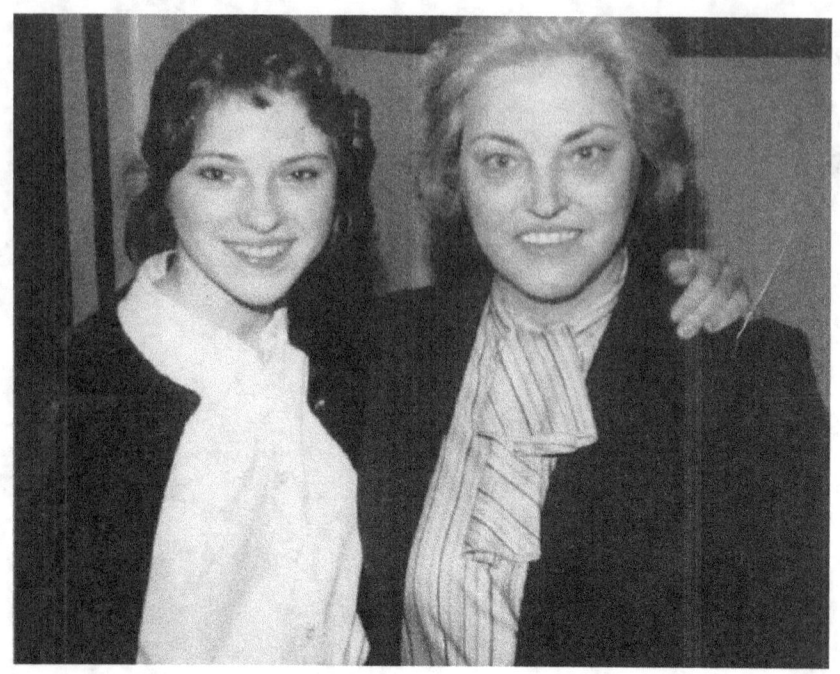

Nancy with her mother.

Chapter 16

After my mother's death, I went back to college and received my bachelor's degree in nursing. I found joy in working with those who suffered, particularly those who struggled with mental illness.

I often reflect on how I prayed all those years that my family would never die. As I have grown older, I have come to realize that even though the people I prayed for have all passed away, my prayers were answered. Today I am the mother of six wonderful children who are honored to have the legacy of a wonderful family, specifically that of an amazing grandmother. When I watch my children meet the challenges of life with courage, I see my mother's influence living on. My mother has taught her family that while we cannot always control what happens to us in this mortal journey, we can always find a way to love.

MY BUTTERFLY

(Written during my college years)

Somewhere inside that wrinkled form
Lies a beauty beyond compare,
A butterfly so rich with life
With so much love to share.

For once she'd fly—oh she could soar
Coloring the world which she knew,
She left a song wherever she went
She left a place anew.

But now she's taken off those wings
And put them far aside,
Instead she's locked in her cocoon,
A home so wrinkled and so dried.

My mother my dear . . . come out, I say
Come out and live with me,
There's so much I want to share with you
So much that we could be.

What happened, Mom, what happened to
the songs you used to sing?
And what about that beauty queen
Who wanted everything?

Your smiles, your goals, your happiness
Have they taken a permanent leave?
Your social wit and intelligence
Are they also beyond retrieve?

You used to travel you used to plan
And how well you wore your face,
Now confusion rings about your soul
And I wonder who has taken your place?

All through your life you saved up clothes
For that "little girl someday,"
And now I'm here and your only child
Oh, won't you come out and play?

We look alike, they tell us both
And how that makes you grin,
Perhaps in me you see the you
You wish you could have been.

It's been so hard to see you ill
Schizophrenia is the label,
But what does that mean to the little girl
Whose mother talks to the table?

Police came often it seemed to me
With handcuffs to take you away,
"Can I go too?" was the little girl's plea
"Stay here with your Grandma," they'd say.

In hospitals you lived dear Mom
So many of those years,
When you were home, I knew you not
For Grandma calmed my fears.

And what about those many times
You'd yell things so insane?
What's Russia got to do with this
And why is Tom Jones to blame?

You'd spit, you'd swear, you'd scream and yell
Or talk softly under your breath,
And always you'd blame someone else
For your seemingly spiritual death.

In the dark I'd hear you get up from bed
And run downstairs so fast,
I'd cuddle to Gram and close my eyes
And wait for the slamming to pass.

But not always were you like this Mom
For at times you were a more puzzling case,
You'd laugh and laugh all day long it seemed
Until you glowed red in the face.

Too much of the time—a pitiful sight
You'd lie on the couch constantly,
Depression made you numb and limp
Rarely could you speak to me.

Eventually I lost my Gram
And you and I were left alone,
I tried so hard to make our house
A warm and happy home.

Today you're as a beaten pup
So lifeless, drained and weak,
You need me for your strength I know
But Mom, so many things I seek.

I love you Mom and I always will
There's so much I want to give,
But not myself—I want to grow
Now it's my turn to live.

Christmas is coming and I'll be home
Right there by your side,
I love serving you with all my heart
And helping your troubled stride.

And one day maybe not in this life
But one coming soon Dear Mother,
You'll put on your wings and fly for me
And we will know each other.

~

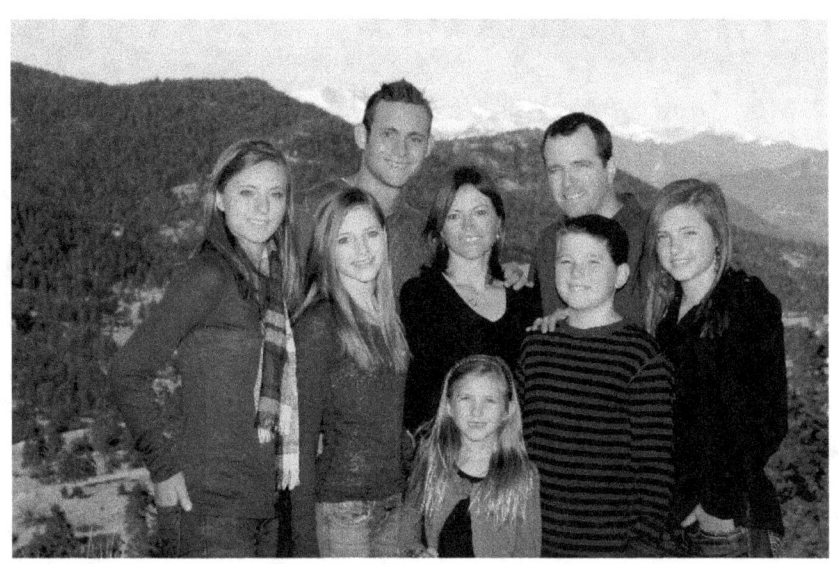

NANCY GRACE WILLIAMSON lives in Colorado with her family. She is the mother of six children. She loves the mountains, skiing, biking, cooking, and, of course, her dogs, Rocky and Bear.